Heart Attack!

Then What?

by Norman Molesko

Heart Attack! Then What?

Copyright © 2011 by Norman Molesko

Printed in the U.S.A.
ISBN: 978-1461034148
Front cover by Sylvia Molesko
Back cover photo by Ellen Tiep www.ellentiep.com
First Edition

DEDICATION

To modern chemistry and technology.

To a host of medical and allied health specialists.

To my loving family and friends.

To all well-wishers.

To my self-determination.

All have enabled me to live on.

PREFACE

This book is about my experiences with coronary heart disease, which often appears as a heart attack. According to the Centers for Disease Control and Prevention, heart disease is the leading cause of death in the United States. In 2009, an estimated 785,000 Americans had an initial heart attack. About 470,000 will have a recurrent attack. Approximately every 25 seconds, an American will have a coronary event and about one every minute will die from one.

In the American Heart Association 2010 Heart & Stroke Statistics, an estimated 81.1 million Americans have one or more types of cardiovascular disease. Of these, 38.1 million are estimated to be age 60 and older.

Social and economic changes contribute to the potential of an even greater numbers of our population becoming affected by heart disease. Influencing factors include: financial insecurity and lifestyle uncertainties; induced personal stresses; unhealthy eating and smoking habits; the explosion of Baby Boomers moving into retirement, many of them with predisposed health conditions; and longer life expectancies for the elderly.

INTRODUCTION

Experience provides the knowledge and intuition which influence how we take care of our health.

This book chronicles my experiences, looking back one year to my first and second heart attacks, seven days apart and what has followed as an aftermath. I capture my thoughts and feelings, as I live through these experiences over time, to reach a state of relative wellness with an usually positive attitude. I reveal to you, another person, what went through my mind and what I felt.

Family, friends, caregivers and people with current heart issues can gain from my knowledge, intuition and positive insights.

ACKNOWLEDGEMENTS

These poems were previously published in my first book, *Retiring And Senior Living, Experiencing The Second Half Of Life:*

"*A Goal For Cholesterol*"
"*It's My Experience*"
"*There's Vroom In Me*"
"*Time Traveler*"
"Won't Power"

Other poems previously published are as follows:

"*Finally...Stenting*"
California Writers Club San Fernando Branch
The Valley Scribe

"*On The Treadmill*"
California Writers Club San Fernando Branch
The Valley Scribe

"*There's Vroom In Me*"
Episcopal Diocese of Maryland *The Gift of Aging*

"*Treasures*"
California Writers Club West Valley Branch
InFocus

"*When My World Changes*"
California Writers Club San Fernando Branch
The Valley Scribe

TABLE OF CONTENTS

IT'S MY EXPERIENCE

I had an experience.

I remembered it.

I told someone about it.

That person didn't have the experience.

That person doubted me.

I know that I had the experience.

It cannot be taken away from me.

The experience belongs to me.

WHEN MY WORLD CHANGES

I swallow a prune, slightly chewed.
Thought the prune would dissolve.
A deep pain in the middle of my chest.
A pressure spot the size of a half dollar.
My left arm feels frail, weak and numb.
I chew four baby aspirins.
I follow up with an antacid pill.
The sensations remain just the same.
I place two nitros under my tongue
about five minutes apart.
I sense no relief to my disbelief.
My thinking is keen, yet in a haze.
I tell my wife to call 911 for help
A few fleeting minutes of waiting.
Six able attendants at my side.
Monitored vital signs recorded.
Answers to questions given.
Telephone conversations heard.
Decisions affecting me are made.
I am in competent care, putting me at ease.
I am placed on a narrow gurney,
moved through open ambulance doors.
I thankfully say,
God bless the 911 team.

MY FIRST HEART ATTACK

I was admitted to an emergency unit of a local hospital. After some testing, I was moved to a bed in a telemetry unit, A few hours later, it was confirmed I was definitely having a heart attack. I was taken on a gurney to an observation unit. Here, early the next day, my groin area was prepared for a heart catheter procedure and whatever else had to be done to save my life. I was taken by ambulance to a second hospital that housed a catheterization laboratory. After an hour wait I was moved and rolled onto their operating table. I was given sedation and underwent an invasive procedure that imaged my heart from inside my body. In somewhat less than an hour, I became conscious. I was informed by a surgeon that I have two clogged artery branches in my heart, both with 95% blockage.

I was told that I would need to take several heart-related medications daily for the rest of my life. In the judgment of the medical team, both heart artery branches were too small to accept a stent emplacement. I stayed on my back with a heavy weight on my groin for three hours and was instructed not to move the right side of my body until the weight was removed.

This was done so that the catheter incision site into the groin-to-heart artery would not start bleeding.

After the procedure, I was transferred back to the first hospital. It was almost an hour ride in the ambulance. I was returned to the same direct observation unit and to the same bed I remembered leaving several hours earlier. I was surprised and thankful that the bed was being held for me until my return. I felt welcomed, being back at this unit. Two days later I was discharged from this hospital and my wife drove me home.

DODGING THE BULLET

(Waiting to be discharged from the hospital
after having the first heart attack)

Smile and more smiles.

I have so many smiles.

This reflects how my soul feels.

It is with a fatigued sense of glee.

The chances could be possible I have found

of being able to stay around

for a future...difficult to foresee.

Lord, I hope you agree that my life should be.

MY SECOND HEART ATTACK

When I arrived home after my first heart attack, I felt several slight intermittent chest sensations and weakness. They continued for the next two days. I woke up for breakfast. I took my morning meds. After the meds, I rested periodically for most of the day. I ate my lunch, dinner and took my meds again. I slept deeply during the nights. During the third day home I was fine. I was taken on a drive and toward the end of the drive, we stopped at a yogurt shop and parked the car rather close to the shop. I carefully selected the best yogurt for me and my heart, non-fat and sugar-free. Eating that dessert was sheer delight. We drove home and I still was fine.

On the morning of the next day, I ate my usual bowl of shredded wheat cereal, milk and a small banana. I had a small additional amount of cereal and milk. I started feeling some chest discomfort. This lasted about four hours. I called an Advice R.N. and was advised to take a nitro, but took an antacid first, sitting up, not lying down. The pain subsided almost fully. I ate a small lunch and a light dinner. I then took my meds, including ½ metoprolol, which made me tired and sleepy. I slept from 6:30 pm to 10:00 pm.

When I awoke, there was some heart discomfort. I became stressed because my wife had an outbreak of diarrhea, vomiting, dizziness and chills for two or three hours. I tried to help her, cleaning up blankets, making tea for her, warming a heating pad when her hands and legs cramped. By that time I was sensing stronger chest pains myself. I took two antacids and four baby aspirins. A few minutes after taking my first nitro, I felt a little better. Next I took my second nitro. My head hurt and I became dizzy. I told my wife, who was by now feeling somewhat better, to call 911. Due to the severity of my heart condition, I was taken to a third close by hospital by ambulance. This hospital had a catheterization laboratory. I was admitted to emergency, hurting a lot. My head was fuzzy again and my memory not clear about what was occurring. All I knew was sharp pain. I was transferred to a cardio-vascular unit and given a battery of tests. I tried to rest. I could not sleep. Eventually I was informed that my Troponin level was critical and I had had a second heart attack.

A FRIGHTENING PERIOD FOR ME AND WIFE

It is during my second heart attack. I am in a bed in a cardio-vascular unit of the third hospital. It is 8:30 in the morning. I am groggy for I have not slept at all during that night. After being moved to this unit, a lady in white re-attaches several electrode patches to my body. From my bed I hear the beeping of my vital signs, coming from a monitor screen The monitor is just behind as well as above my head. I cannot see the screen. Oxygen silently flows into my nostrils. My left thumb is immobile and uncomfortable, due to the stiff splint firmly taped to my wrist. The splint secures the needle into my vein and connects at the other end to a plastic I.V. tube. A cotton sheet and wool blanket are draped over my body and my pain-laden chest.

My mind plays one theme. I feel I am reaching the end of my existence. A flow of sounds, cries and words escapes from my lips to my wife. She is seated in a chair near the bed. She listens with tenderness and jots down some of my thoughts on a yellow pad. I try to communicate what I feel will be needed to be done before and after I pass on. I have streams of fleeting thoughts. Suddenly I begin sobbing uncontrollably. I am full of fear. I do not want to die, but I am convinced I am going to. My wife tries to voice reassurance, but I am totally absorbed in myself. It must be heart-wrenching for her to witness.

FINALLY...STENTING

Two days lying in one hospital,
then being transferred to another hospital.
A RN accompanies me in an ambulance.
I become bewildered and scared.

I feel that I am on the brink of death...
a second traumatic attack in seven days.
The culprit for this second attack
is the occlusion in my first diagonal artery,
that is almost entirely blocked in my heart.

For each of the two separate heart attacks,
as I am "going under" on the operating table,
I put myself into a pliable state of mind.
My body is a piece of willing wood...
carve and do what you want to save me!

After my first heart invasive procedure, I am told
that medications are my regular treatment.
After the second heart invasive procedure, I sensed
the one stent emplacement was challenging to do.

I am fortunate that the stent emplacement
is a reprieve, allowing me to keep on living.
I hope many breaths can put off my death.
I don't want to leave and have folks grieve.

MY CLAIM

I am born and
evolve to where I am.
My claim to life is that
I am here...now.

INCREDIBLE

It's today.

A MIRACLE

Second by second, moment by moment,
another cycle of lub-dub, lub-dub, lub-dub,
as my heart rate keeps beating on
and my soul lingers with life.

WHERE I NEED TO BE

At home, after my second heart attack,
I presume I am holding my own
but with fragility and uncertainty.

Alone. No hustling.
Solitude and quiet
allow me to mend and recover.

Time silently witnesses
the ebb and flow of my life.
After distressing episodes,
streams of soothing music
slowly drift in and out
of the pores of my soul.
This is where I need to be,
calm and serene,
away from any storm.

FEELINGS ABOUT OTHERS

I am comfortable with folks

who say one thing and follow through,

not say one thing and then do another.

I appreciate those who are consistent

and always candid with me.

CONCERNS BY OTHERS

People have offered advice…well-intentioned.

I can be captured by the influence of others.

I have to allow myself the freedom

to back away from this advice.

I have to exert self-determination

to stand clear from such influences,

not dismissing them from consideration.

My own inherent abilities are ever-present.

I need to think for myself to be in control

whenever my brain is alert and ready.

I cannot rely on the best intentions of others,

for these may not be what is best for me.

YOU WANT TO KNOW HOW I FEEL?

I sit and contemplate why I am I here.
Reason and thought come and go.
I grasp onto one and follow it where it leads.
If it becomes irrelevant, I take another path.

Some days are better than others, I guess.
I am physically rather weak…positive or glum.
Persons living through similar experiences
may know and connect with how I feel.

I realize I am tending to be egocentric,
preoccupied even more so with myself,
but in a sense isn't everyone like this…
in a reality of their very own?

A CONTINUAL CHALLENGE

The human make-up allows us
to have an openness and close-up
of oneself in our universe,
to observe, understand, empathize,
to have scope and cope.

After a heart attack or illness,
I don't drive myself,
don't be a runabout,
don't push, push, push…
give myself leeway.

I cut down to a minimum,
avoid situations causing anxiety,
allow myself to mend,
don't wear myself out.
I stop…before becoming a dropout.

I hope family and friends are aware
my heart can act up at times.
I have to cater to its calling.

WHAT TO DO NEXT?

Hey! You down there!
came a voice from above.
You claim you are suffering
with post heart attack blues,
an ache, a twinge, a spasm,
a shadow feeling of phantom hurt.
You say the discomfort in your chest area
is difficult to describe, to pinpoint.
Could it possibly be angina or heartburn?
Is it brief, lingers on or goes away?
You have to choose for yourself what to do.
Ignore, tolerate, reach out for advice,
take antacids, low dose aspirins, nitro,
call 911 for an emergency ambulance.
Another important thing to remember…
hope is offered from above.

WITHIN MY CAPABILITIES

A few signposts are given to me
to indicate which lifestyle I should echo.
I must start off slow and easy,
minute by minute, hour by hour.
I increase my activities,
following the sensible advice
given by my cardiologist.

I am incapable of doing things on-the-run,
as in former years I would have done.
I don't want to view my life as ticking away.
When some project becomes overwhelming,
I have to moderate my expectations.
I need patience to wait and postpone activities
to a time more fitting and appropriate.

I don't anticipate climbing a mountain.
In my situation, I am practical and a realist.

MY SPASM SENSATION

Something awful is happening,

a cramp in an upper body muscle of mine,

a contraction, an ache, a pain.

I'm in my own chasm…sensing this spasm.

It's hurting. It's excruciating.

I place a heating pad in a micro-wave.

Waiting for the pad to heat up, I rave and rave.

Then…I apply some heat to the muscle.

Finally…the warmth with its relaxing relief

steals away from my mind the prior grief.

BEING MORE SELF-SUFFICIENT

Maybe yes, maybe no.

I show acceptance.

I have denial.

I wear a happy smile.

I have doubt.

I revel in being alive.

I may feel sad.

So much to adjust to.

All could not be anticipated.

There are many things to handle

that could easily lead to confusion.

I must not become besieged.

Over these past weeks of adjustments,

my life settles down somewhat.

I am being more self-sufficient.

I don't hope to repeat what I went through.

PRIVILEGED WITH LIFE

While I am gradually recovering,

I feel another setback.

Another disappointment.

Yet I keep on living,

not oblivious to the bumps.

This is the way I am.

I get into a frame of mind

to put on a pleasant face.

I am thankful for what I possess.

I can stand up and stretch.

KEEPING THE HEART BEATING

I haven't forgotten both heart attacks, not one,
and the emplacement of a coronary artery stent.
Not all chest discomfort have gone away.
It is several weeks since that surgery day.

Referring to all the details I have to handle,
my initial tasks were viewed at times as hectic.
Body sensations and stress lead me to be uptight.
I have found effective ways to feel all right.

I now live within additional confines,
meds, diet, exercise and non-mentionable things.
I don't re-touch such life-sustaining requirements.
I do what I have to do to manage all.

I trust my medications are a must for me.
The health of my heart should be OK, on-par.
My mainstay is a brew of metoprolol, pepcid,
plavix, aspirin, isosorbide, zocor and cozaar.

Rehab will add to this life-sustaining brew.
With a plan for 36 monitored exercise sessions,
I expect to strengthen my body and my heart.
The right diet remains a necessary counter-part.

And my heart keeps beating.

LOCATING MY PILLS

I am taking seven heart pills.
I put them down somewhere.
I don't know where I place them.
They are critical life-giving pills.
My forgetting is getting worse.

For health-care reasons there is the necessity
to better organize my pills and refills,
no cubbyholes and odd spaces I go to in haste.
A pill box organizer houses them in a fitting place.
The organizer aids me in taking pills systematically.

WON'T POWER

I have become discreet about what I eat.

Generally I'm in the right mindset.

about my selection of food.

I don't have to fret.

Some people devour almost anything,

any time, at any hour of the day.

They say I WILL have some.

That is WILL POWER.

Somehow, I can empower myself,

to avoid eating just anything, anytime.

I can say I WON'T have any.

That is WON'T POWER.

A GOAL FOR CHOLESTEROL

Cholesterol can be nutritious.

A jelly roll can be delicious.

Some folks intake cholesterol often

in a manner quite capricious.

About my health and cholesterol,

I must be careful about both.

High cholesterol intake is harmful.

This is fact for me, not fictitious.

How much cholesterol do I intake,

while being careful to moderate?

At home and in a restaurant,

my goal is to remain judicious.

WATER IS BENEFICIAL

I have started to love water.

Drink two quarts a day.

Take some before I eat.

It keeps me hydrated.

It dissolves my meds.

A natural liquid, so neat.

I love water.

Use it to shower.

Cool the body.

Clean the feet.

Rinse the teeth.

It becomes a treat.

I love water.

It helps when tense.

Clears the head when dense.

Its benefits are immense.

Respecting what it does

makes good sense.

TREASURES

Sensing relief from discomfort is a simple pleasure.
For me, each simple pleasure is really treasured.

Feeling chilled on a wintry day,
trembling, cold down to the bones,
then sipping hot soup is so warming. Ahh!

Having a splitting headache,
with agonizing pain in the brain,
then the migraine is not there. Ahh!

A cramping in the upper leg,
causing anguish and screaming,
then the pain stops. Ahh!

Being blasted by raucous music,
assaulting to the ears,
then the noise abruptly stops. Ahh!

I can go on and on, but what I mean to say is
when a feeling of discomfort leaves me any day,
Ahh!, this sense of relief is indeed a pleasure,
though noticed only for a moment or two.

I hold such moments as precious,
valuing each as being a treasure.
Certainly you must have collected
many of these treasures during your lifetime.

PRAISING MY BEING

I know I am a normal fellow,
made up of flesh and blood,
my body directed more by my mind.
It's like that for most mankind.

I mumble at times
about the mundane,
yet should I take
my life for granted?

I can wander around
within my comfort zone.
I would not be pleased
to scram from where I am.

I comprehend
how vulnerable my existence is,
not with fear, but wholesome cheer.
I am alive and active here.

A GOOD QUALITY OF LIFE

I'm emotionally alive, not emotionally dead.

You should understand that. It's what I said.

I'm involved in life. Not withdrawn.

I wake up. Open my eyes. It's a fine day.

The day is swell because I feel well.

I'm living. I'm vital. I've been given extra time.

I can enjoy, appreciate and celebrate.

When I'm engaged in creative endeavors,

I cease being absorbed with cardiac concerns.

I've learned to balance what I do.

Such acts allow me to realize my true self

and add enrichment to my life.

EXERCISING WITH PERSISTENCE

I was strongly urged by a physical therapist

to sign into a customized cardiac rehab program.

My cardiologist consented when my body was ready.

Near the beginning of rehab, I experienced some distress.

I clenched my fists, gritted my teeth, determined to go on.

I didn't complain, stumble nor succumb to self-pity.

Now that I am further along with my rehab sessions,

I often pat myself on the back with feelings of success.

It's my way to provide myself positive feedback.

I feel fortunate for this opportunity to mend my heart.

POSITIVE IMAGERY

I started my rehab session program,

able to concentrate on exercising

with the abilities I have remaining.

Positive thinking is how my mind is cast,

taking on some challenges as they arise,

but wise enough not to fall for lies.

During my earlier sessions…

Ouch! Ouch! Ouch!

Chest muscles really hurt.

I drop onto my living room couch.

The discomfort I had

eventually dissipates.

Following my third week of sessions…

my attitude and outlook,

Calm! Calm! Calm!

Chest muscles sense no harm.

I sit upon the same couch

and hum a cheerful tune.

I AWOKE TO MIND AND BODY

I had always been a *head* person,

not oriented toward body-building.

Now exercise has become *vital* to my existence.

Each fitness machine energizes me,

helping me gain a new lease on life.

I am a fitness activist, a new enthusiast.

My previous lifestyle was *mind first*.

My body, however, took second place.

Now *mind and body* are on *equal footing*.

What a difference in my quality of life!

Get up. Move around. Don't be sedentary.

I can think thoughts of love and charm,

but that doesn't help my body stay fit.

I require regular physical activity.

It's for my health. I can't forget it.

AN ANNOYANCE

If I experience an annoyance
which seems small or large,
I may shrug and try to ignore it.
I can say to myself,
it is only an external thing.
It doesn't really matter.
I don't care. I wish to let it go.
Yet there must be other ways to cope.

Employ a technique
to relax the mind.
Breathe slowly in and out,
meditate with tranquility.
Then think about what to do,
consider the matter wisely.
Take action and follow through
and let it go…let it go.

LAUGHTER AND SMILING

Life can become too serious,

so I mingle with joyful feelings.

I sprinkle seriousness with pleasure.

I look up and the stars twinkle.

I become aware of bells jingling.

Life lingers on with pleasure.

If I don't ever laugh,

I might be uptight.

If I don't ever smile,

life would be dreary.

I indulge in laughter and smiling,

keeping healthy with happiness.

MY EXERCISE PALS

In this rehab playground,
I have grown to love the dynamic machines.
Each day they awaken when I arrive.
Every one is ready to become active, alive.

A few weeks after the start of my rehab program,
these machines have bonded with me.
The aerobic and resistance machines
allow me to exercise my imagination.

The treadmill is thrilled when I walk on it.
The bicycle is delighted as I treadle its pedals.
The leg press sighs, pleased as I push in and out.
The ergometer is aroused when my hands clasp it.

I ready my muscles and heart.
The experts tell me I will be healthier to persist.
The attending nurses are read on the spot.
They are all helpful, caring and know a lot.

ON THE TREADMILL

I stretch. I warm up.
I chat to my machine, my friend.
I set my walking speed. And reset.
Need more speed. Some more.
To mend, to strengthen. I sing,
Go higher. Go higher. Go higher.
I'm on fire.
Go higher. Go higher. Go higher.
I'm working harder.
Go higher. Go higher. Go higher.
My numbers are increasing for the better.
My body wants it faster.
Increase the elevation, elevate the speed.
Then I feel twinges in the middle of my chest.
Is it my heart or another muscle in arrest?
Go moderate. Go lower.
My mind tells me slower.
I have been easily carried away
by too much momentum.
I realize I have to slow down
to a lower speed I can handle.
It is time for me to adjust and drop down.

BIKING IS FITNESS FUN

I'm straddling the reclining bike,
starting off with setting speed and time.
I have grown to care for this machine
and this machine cares for me too,
like a cowboy bonding with his horse.

Our activities begin with legs and knees.
My right knee goes down, the left knee up.
The knees move up and down and around.
I talk kindly to this health aiding machine.
It hums back to me during our routine.

I have fun on this bike of mine,
the magic, the rhythm, the moving pace.
I know in my head not to ride too high.
I keep on peddling along
and smile to those passing by.

IS THIS THE LEG PRESS? YES!

I decide on a weight and add this to the press.

I sit down on the seat and tilt it back a bit.

Adjust the seat for the distance to my feet.

Place my shoes upon the footplates. No big feat.

I slowly exhale with my legs angled and bent.

My legs push downward with force, away from me.

I allow the air in my lungs to breathe out.

The angle made by my legs is almost straight.

Then I slowly begin to inhale in, filling up my lungs.

My legs move in reverse from before, becoming angled.

This releases the leg tension that has been built up.

I keep on exhaling out, inhaling in for each press cycle.

If I push down and then release the pressure on this machine.

I should find it easier at home to raise myself from a soft chair.

THEY CALL IT THE ARM ERGOMETER

The ergometer is a bicycle using the arms and hands.
Both hands grasp and rotate a wheel showing resistance.
One hand goes forward…up, the other backward…down.
With my body I can swivel to the left and right for fun.

This is a machine for upper body development,
for lifting, throwing, swimming, reaching.
I have tolerated periods of transient discomfort,
but the effort makes me feel stronger and better.

SELF-PRESERVATION IS ON THE LINE

My mood is in good spirits nowadays,

months after my cardiac bouts.

I am in much better physical shape.

My morale is high without any doubt.

Yet...I do not idealize my situation.

I realize how quickly things can change.

Most people may not think about it,

but sudden twists in life do exist.

I show allegiance to self-preservation,

as I move off into the world of today, alive.

A few more drinks. A few more eats.

A few more breaths. A few more beats.

TIME WHIZZES BY

Time doesn't rest.
Time doesn't pause.
When I am busy,
time zooms by.

Everything takes time,
anytime I think,
anytime I speak,
anytime I do anything.

Saying one, two, three,
this takes three seconds.
I shouldn't look surprised
nor raise an eyebrow.

Time is like a spark
I can reflect about it and remark,
time doesn't holdfast.
Time moves like a photoflash.

THERE'S VROOM IN ME

I've turned on the ignition,
put my car into drive,
took my foot off the brake,
stepped on the gas.

My car barely started
with a putt, putt, putt,
picked up some oomph,
zoomed ahead with a vroom.

Several days later I had begun
to garden under the summer sun.
I became weak and exhausted.
I lost my vroom.

Deep within my chest,
my breathing was labored,
as when my car went
putt, putt, putt.

I sat down to rest awhile,
drank a pint of water,
and waited around patiently
for my vroom to resume.

A SCARE AND A LESSON LEARNED

I think I am brave and I can do.

I have completed 36 rehab sessions,

feeling mentally and physically fit.

With masculine bravado I am demonstrating

proudly to my wife, that I can lift and carry

a full package of 24 one-pint water bottles,

from a shopping cart into the trunk of our car.

Wrong! What I did in earlier days of yore,

I should not still try to do now as I did before.

Two hours after this bravado feat, it hit me again,

with chest pains going from slight to moderate.

I become scared, felt dependent and helpless.

I did what I had to do to respond to the pain.

The pain subsided after a relatively long time.

I must be careful not to lift and carry heavy things.

TIME TRAVELER

My life span can be depicted

by a straight-edge of unknown length.

I am a senior time traveler

moving along a ruler's edge.

Markings on the strip reveal

the events that have come and gone.

I know where I am on the strip

but don't know where the ruler ends.

No concern about frailty.

No dependence on strength.

No prediction of longevity.

There are no immediacies to send

any thoughts back to the past.

No need to cast any glances ahead

to a future of uncertainty and unknown.

I am alive in this twinkling of a second.

Each second belongs to me as my own.

RESPECTING LIFE

I have been pondering about this.
I avoid drifting toward a mental abyss.
No longer can I further resist.
I need to tell you now what for me exists.

When I focus about the time ahead,
today I will be living one day less.
When I think about time since I was born,
today I will be living one day more.

Like many folks who are aging,
I glance forward and glimpse backward.
I reflect on life and what I know now.
I respect life to its core.

ALWAYS A HEART PATIENT

I'll always be a heart patient.
I'm now active, happy and sane.
It's twelve months since my attacks,
since I escaped the guillotine of death.
These are candid feelings.

So I take my meds
as the doctor says,
eat right and exercise,
do my best to pass all lab tests,
try to minimize risks and be wise.

I'm able to live a good life.
though I will remain a heart patient
for the rest of my days.

ABOUT THE AUTHOR

Norman Molesko was trained as a psychologist. He has served as a psychologist and nursing home administrator and human factors specialist. He has been on the Council on Aging with the Los Angeles City Department of Aging. The author's poems show knowledge, intuition and positive insights on Senior and Health issues. The poems communicate, inform and connect.

His two published books are *Retiring And Senior Living, Experiencing The Second Half Of Life* and *Heart Attack! Then What?*

Two of his poems for patients are being displayed at the Cardiac Rehabilitation and Fitness Center at the Valley Presbyterian Hospital, the Department of Cardiology at the Kaiser Permanente Woodland Hills Medical Center, the Department of Audiology at the Kaiser Permanente Panorama City Medical Center and at the HearX Facility in Reseda, California.

He is "Poet Laureate" for the California Retired Teachers Association, San Fernando Valley Division, and "Resident Poet" of the *Valley Voice* Newspaper. He was named "Featured Writer of the Month" by the Senior Citizens Section, Los Angeles Dept. of Recreation & Parks in July 2009. Norman was the featured poet at the Senior Talent Show for the 2009 Los Angeles Dept. of Aging *Celebration of Older Americans Month*.

His poems have also appeared in the Gerontological Society of America *Journal of Aging, Humanities and the Arts*, Valley Voice Newspaper, Pierce College *ENCORE Older Adult News,* Episcopal Diocese of Maryland *Gift of Aging*, Wilkinson Multipurpose Senior Center Newsletter, California Senior Legislature Newsletter, California Writers Club *Valley Scribe* and *In/Focus* Newsletters, the Los Angeles Dept. of Recreation & Parks *Senior Moments* and on the rthridge 100 website and the Halifax Canada Chronic Pain Support Group website.